Wellbeing-
Pure & Simple!

Nic Hartshorne

ISBN: 9781798464175

DEDICATION

To my dear Flynn- who taught me so much.

CONTENTS

PREFACE

PREFACE

WELLBEING – PURE & SIMPLE!

Forgive me, but there is a slight irony in the title, I wanted to write a short book that helped people to live a more fulfilling life, where they felt mentally well and had well-being. After working within health and wellbeing for over 20 years, I know it is not that simple- or is it.......?

I hope you will find this book accessible, thought provoking and stimulating. My target audience is anyone who is interested in a holistic view of health, whether you've been exploring this stuff for years, or whether you're dipping your toe in.

So, what do I mean by holistic – to me holistic means a sense of the whole, the dictionary definition is 'all-inclusive and rounded.' It is my belief that we are made up of a mind, body, spirit dimension and all these parts must be heard and acknowledged at some level.

The book will not tell you how to achieve your own sense of wellbeing – that is for you to work out, but there may be certain bits of the book that resonate with you more than others -we are all unique and on our own journey and at different times in our lives we may need to pay attention to different things.

Nor, does the book promise to be a magic panacea for wellness, but instead I hope we can together explore a few ideas about this 'stuff.' By exploring these ideas together, my belief is, that everything is relational, so although we are not in the same room or indeed I do not know you, by reading this we are having a conversation, you will digest the words and make your own unique sense of what I'm saying and it will have unique meaning to *you* -just as if we were having a 'real conversation.'

Let us begin….

1 WHAT IS MENTAL HEALTH AND WELLBEING?

During my time working in the National Health Service, I became aware quite quickly that people feared the term mental health, I think it conjured up images of the asylums of the past, that indeed existed and some people had personal experience of relatives being placed there. However, my idea of mental health is the notion that actually we **all** have mental health, it isn't something that happens to us when we are distressed, or only a few have mental health, we **all** have health. People seem much more comfortable with thinking about the term physical health, we understand that, we know we must eat in order to survive, we know we need to have water in order to survive, we know if we eat healthier foods it is better for us, we know we should combine this with some sort of physical exercise in order to be healthier- yes- sound familiar, we've all heard this stuff. But what of mental health, how much energy, or indeed thought do we put into keeping mentally well?

 According to the World health organization 'Health is a state of complete physical, mental and social well-being and not merely the absence of disease or infirmity.' Let's take a few minutes to think about the enormity of the task at hand……, it will indeed take a deliberate effort on our part to service the needs of all the different components. However, as has been eluded to earlier, the focus of this book is to draw our attention to the specific element called, 'mental health'.

My take on why people seem to struggle with the idea of mental health is that we can't see it, when it's not working as well as it might be it doesn't show up on an X ray! But at times, part of the human condition is to feel emotional pain, yes actually *feel t*he pain, just as if we had experienced a blow or physical attack on our body and at times the pain feels intolerable to the point that we want the suffering to end and the only conceivable way we can imagine it ending, is to die……, that's quite a sobering thought, I feel, but true.

So, if that isn't a good reason to pay attention to our emotional needs, I don't know what is.

According to Carl Rogers the founder of person centered therapy, given the right conditions human beings can flourish. Let's spend some time exploring together some of the components that could make up the 'right' conditions……

2 THE SCIENCE OF KINDNESS

You only have to do an internet search on the effects of kindness to see that there have been numerous studies demonstrating that being kind, doing a kind deed, or saying something kind can release chemicals in the brain to make us feel good. That sounds pretty win- win in my book! And I would highly recommend giving it a go… go on what have you got to lose? It doesn't have to be big, I'd even go as far as saying just smiling, yes smiling at someone as you walk past can have an effect. For most of us life can be pretty hectic, or for some maybe not busy enough, but whatever, a simple act of kindness can go a long way.

This brings me onto the main purpose for this chapter, which is about kindness, *but* as well as being kind to others, when was the last time you were kind to yourself?

I'm always amazed at how pretty unkind us humans can be to ourselves at times. I think this can be demonstrated in an overt way, or can be incredibly subtle, I've listed a few of the ways that I've come across over the years of how people have not been kind to themselves, myself included! I think many of us don't deliberately set out to be unkind, but it's not until we think about it, I mean really think about it, that we realise we are doing it, here are some examples below:

- Over eating, how many of us are actually in touch with that part of us that says, 'I'm full'…., most of us eat whilst on automatic pilot.

- Eating foods, we know are unhealthy for us

- Not eating enough wholesome nourishing food

- Drinking too much alcohol

- Not drinking enough water

- Over exercising

- Not exercising enough (even going for a short walk is exercise!)

- Not going to that Yoga class when we know we always feel better afterwards!

- Talking to ourselves in an abusive way, (Sometimes these are introjects we've heard from other people.)

- Working too much,

- Staying in a job that doesn't fulfil us

- Not working enough, or doing something purposeful

- Not slowing or stopping to appreciate the…………… (fill in the gaps)

- Not attending to our personal hygiene in a kind way by not nurturing our bodies. We

can have a bath, or shower, or we can
have a bath or shower in a way that is
done with kindness

- Denying ourselves meaningful
  relationships with others

- Allowing ourselves to be abused by others

- Not allowing ourselves to make mistakes

- Not trying new things

- Not having fun

- Thinking that you don't deserve to
  experience happiness, satisfaction,
  contentment etc.

- Not being in nature

- Not paying attention to *your* needs

I'm sure there are more…. but do you get the
picture, that it's not always that obvious, in the
way we deny ourselves kindness.

I think particularly in western society many of us are under the notion that being kind to ourselves, thinking about what we need or want is selfish, but I believe it's the opposite, It's imperative we are kind to ourselves.

One of my favorite sayings is

'You can't pour from an empty cup….'

I'd like you just to spend some time thinking about what you can do to be kinder to yourself, for some of you that may not come easy, for others, you may think that you *are* kind to yourself, so the ways you aren't kind may be less overt, but I bet there is something on the list that you would benefit from doing more, or less of….

Please don't get me wrong this isn't meant to send you on a guilt trip because you haven't been kind! Instead it's just about encouraging you to begin to let go- shrug your shoulders- loosen the tension and start to build a loving relationship with yourself……

3 A RELATIONAL NARRATIVE

Where did I learn to not love myself? I don't want to spend hours analyzing this, but I think it's safe to say, we all have introjects, voices that we've internalised over the years, that we turn into a story, that story can then sometimes turn into our truth.

I'm not worthy, I'm not loveable, I'm not good enough, I'm a bad person, I'm a bad Mother/Father, I'm boring I'm a victim,, blah, blah, blah …..I don't want to make light of introjects, but what I'd like you to consider is they are just stories, stories, thoughts, -I know you're probably screaming at me now, saying but they feel real, they hurt, they're painful!

And I'm not going to argue with you there, but what I'd like to invite you to do is to consider writing some new stories and have a little fun, imagining how it would be to play with the new scripts you could write for yourself. What would you act like if you were this person, what would you wear, how would your posture be, what would you sound like, what would you be doing differently. Maybe today is the day you could try out what it would be like to be this person…?

In the first part of the book we have considered the idea of self- care and the relationship we have with ourselves, which can be known as intra personal, I'd like to now invite you to think about the relationships we have with others, interpersonal.

In the words of the metaphysical poet, John Donne 'no man is an island…'

There is much evidence to suggest that as human beings, to support our wellbeing we need to feel connected. For the purposes of this chapter I'm going to focus on our connection with other human beings.

I'd like you to consider giving some thought to the people in your life, some people at this point find it useful to write down who are the main characters in your life;

Where are they in relation to you, are they where you want them to be?

Do you want to feel closer to them?

Do you want them to be further away?

Are there enough people in your life?

Are there too many?

Are there enough of the right kind of people, by this I mean people on your wavelength?

People who can provide you with practical support?

Remember, this isn't probably going to be just one person, it would be unusual if one person could fulfill all our needs, and if they did, what would happen if they suddenly weren't there?

The central theme in interpersonal therapy suggests the relationships we have with others can have a direct impact on our mood. Have you ever noticed that when you spend time with certain people you feel good, energised, inspired, happier and there are also certain people who can leave you feeling drained, upset or angry. Sometimes people can even project their stuff onto us.

For whatever reason some relationships don't work for us. Remember we're all unique and we're not always going to get along with everyone we meet, or feel that connection with everyone- and that's O.K.

I guess the trick is to notice how we feel when we're with other people, be curious about those feelings and notice what they mean to you.

Sometimes relationships that don't work for us are easy not to pursue, because of the context of the relationship, other times it's more tricky, when it's a family member, or work colleague, or a friend, it could be you're friends with that person because you've known them forever, but actually you've both changed and no longer have as much in common, or it could even be your partner.

So, if we consider the theory underpinning interpersonal therapy, that the quality of our relationships can have a direct impact on our mental health and wellbeing, then our relationships and spending time with the right people, is key!

In good relationships it works when, all parties needs have equal priority, which means there may be some negotiation that needs to take place. I think maintaining respectful relationships is the crux of things here, and underpins the philosophy of assertiveness, the idea that we all matter, including ourselves!

I think this concept can at times get a little lost in translation, so on a basic level;

If we are **passive** – we don't value our needs, we feel other people's needs, thoughts, feelings and beliefs are more important than ours.

If we are **aggressive** – we value our needs, thoughts, feelings and beliefs, however, we value them over everyone else's and have little respect for the other.

If we are **assertive** – We value our needs, thoughts, feelings and beliefs and we also value, the needs, thoughts, feelings and beliefs of the other.

Eric Berne famously wrote a book entitled – 'I'm O.K- You're OK.' To me, this short snappy title encapsulates the sentiment in its entirety.

Although I think we've probably all heard of assertiveness, to maintain a true homeostasis, it's perhaps not as easy as it sounds.

It relies on being able to, firstly believe that it's O.K, for us to allow ourselves to have needs, thoughts, feelings and beliefs and secondly to express them in relationship, in a way that treats the other with the same value.

A good way to start in a given situation, is to feel able to say, this is what I think, believe, feel- how about You? If it is similar then great, if not as we said earlier, it may be at this point we need to listen intently to the other and then have a conversation around how we can proceed, that feels acceptable for both parties. Give it a go? A word of advice though, both parties have got to be willing to engage in this way of relating, otherwise you may just end up feeling resentful if you're the one having to deny what's right for you all the time. Also, as I mentioned earlier some relationships are easier not to pursue, depending on the relationship.

So, just another point of clarification, by relationships with others, I'm not making any distinction between which relationships. Assertiveness is more about a philosophy around a way of being, so the intent behind any interaction is coming from the place of 'I value myself and I value you.' So, whether this is with an intimate partner, or the woman in the supermarket, the same could apply. It's about open, honest communication from the intent of respect and a motivation to be a worthy one.

In other words-, saying to someone,' I think you look hideous in that dress', might be true for you, but actually what was the intention or motivation behind that statement, what did you want to achieve by saying it? It certainly doesn't feel like it's coming from a good place!

You may be waking up to the fact for the first time that it's O.K to have needs, thoughts, feelings and beliefs and want to start to

exercise those. However, the road ahead may
not be an easy one and may lead to pain,
particularly if the relationship you want to
explore has been, a kind of symbiotic one
where you've been the one taking care of the
other, to the exclusion of you and the other
person, somewhat understandably, they may
not what you to change.

4 EAST MEETS WEST BEYOND THE REALM……

During the next chapter, I'd like us to consider the subject of spirituality. For some of you that will excite you, for some of you that will scare you, for some of you that will conjure up ideas around religion, and no doubt many other feelings, or thoughts will be evoked.

Over the years I've noticed, perhaps spirituality is the thing that I feel people deny themselves of, more than any other, that spiritual dimension of themselves. But remember, if we are to look at ourselves as holistic beings, I firmly believe spirituality should be included.

What do I mean by spirituality? That's a good question, it's perhaps easier for me to start with, for the purposes of this book, what it isn't.

We're not going to discuss communicating with dead people, or ghosts etc.

We're not going to be talking specifically about religious dogma.

What spirituality means to me, is that deep feeling within, that part of ourselves, perhaps known as the soul, the very essence that helps us explore – 'who am I?'

Donald Winnicott an American Psychiatrist, introduced us to a concept of the false self-versus the true self. When I think about this I imagine the 'true self' to be our soul, what drives us from a heart place rather than a head place. In other words what *feels* right, opposed to what we *think* is right. I hope that makes sense, if you're not accustomed to tuning into your feelings, give it a go, notice how you feel in certain situations. Do you sometimes have a conflict when making decisions choosing between what your heart is saying, opposed to your head? It can be confusing at times. But the suggestion is when we deeply listen through meditation or stillness, that's when we kind of know what's the right answer.

I also think it's that connection we have with something bigger than ourselves, now that, I believe is a very personal and intimate thing.

It could mean a relationship with God and depending if you are religious and the beliefs of that religion, the word God will mean something different.

It could mean the relationship you have with the cosmos, or universe.

It could mean the relationship you have with nature.

It could be your philosophy, take on life, for example believing in fate, or synchronicity.

Although discussing spirituality, particularly certain eastern beliefs, was once thought of esoteric, it is however my experience, that much more the eastern traditions around health and wellbeing are becoming more mainstream.

Examples of such are Yoga, mindfulness, sound healing, tai chi and even shamanism.

If take yoga for example, in a nutshell the process of yoga is to bring us more in touch with our true nature, our essence in the purest sense of the word. Within this process it helps us to 'wake up' and become aware of not only our selves but our environment and how we conduct ourselves in that environment. In other words how 'mindful' are we of our everyday actions and how present we are, as I mentioned earlier, many of us go round on automatic pilot, rushing from here to there, a good example of not being in the present can be when we are driving somewhere, we arrive at our destination and then suddenly think, hang on, how did I get here…. We were thinking about everything but the task in hand, we weren't enjoying the moment.

I'd like you to think about it as you sit here now, think about how comfortable you are in your position, are you tense…. just notice…… mentally scan your body…you may want to adjust things so that you feel more supported and can enjoy the experience of relaxing and reading, rather, than thinking – 'I just need to get through this book to the end, so I can move onto the next book, task' ,or whatever……

Take a few moments to take some deep breaths - inhale through your nose, hold the breath for three, then slowly exhale through the nose, if it's safe to do so deepen the breath each time, really breathing from your stomach, expanding the abdomen rather than your upper chest. Many of spend most of our time using shallow breaths from the upper part of our chest, which at best isn't utilising our body to its maximum potential, at worst it can increase our anxiety or feelings of panic.

I'd encourage you to practice bringing your focus back to the present moment throughout the day, without any judgment, but just try staying with the present moment as much as you can. If in the awareness of the present moment you feel uncomfortable, (obviously if the pain persists or is intense please consult your doctor –I'm talking more of the tensions, aches or uncomfortableness most of us experience from time to time) just notice and try to stay with it using your breath, you may want to just move your body slightly to let go of any tension, just moving the shoulders, or gently shrugging them. We can hold much tension and emotion in our bodies.

It is said that the tradition of yoga dates back over 40,000 years, but within the west it is currently gaining in popularity, perhaps as an antidote to modern western living, where we are constantly stimulated using television, radio, ipads, computers, mobile phones, x box's etc. These are all useful or entertaining, but there is just too much of it for our us to cope with and these are just our wind down activities! We work longer hours and have less and less time to just be.

According to Patanjali's Sutras the process of yoga is focused on the need to control the modifications or waves of the mind. The mind is considered the link between body spirit and consciousness.

Believing the main function of yoga is to help calm the mind in order for a clear perception of what is real and what is false to emerge.

So, whereas western psychology, even though the word 'psychology' means the study of the soul, it has tended to focus on the brain, our thoughts, our sense of self also known as our ego strength, Eastern spirituality is perhaps more multi-layered also encompassing that which is outside ourselves. But also paying attention to our physical body (although there has been a recognition that trauma can reside in the body, talking therapies have mostly been concerned with the head, or feelings, but not particularly the body. With some exceptions to this)   There is an understanding in yoga, speaking particularly about Raja yoga, just because that's the one I have most personal experience with, that emotions can be stored in the body, in our cells and in our tissues.

Therefore, if we are to consider a holistic way of thinking about health, we also need to tend, nurture and heal our bodies. Within Yoga, the belief is that as we move and stretch or bodies in a certain way we are recalibrating and working to reset old and unhelpful patterns.

Again, sound healing and shamanism as alluded to earlier, where although perhaps once thought of as slightly weird,   the benefits of both approaches are becoming more and more apparent and healing us on a more spiritual level. I won't elaborate on either of these approaches, but if you're interested, I would recommend doing some research and finding out more, maybe even attending a session.

5 DRAWING TO A CONCLUSION....

In this Chapter I would like us to consider and reflect upon what we have read in this book and what it means to us, which bits spoke to us directly and resonated at some level?

You may have picked up on a theme that has run throughout the book, which is that of relationships. I said at the beginning of the book that I see the world through the lens of relationships.

The relationship we have with ourselves, including how kind or unkind we are to ourselves, the relationship we have with others, I specifically talked about human beings, but it can include the relationships we have with our animals. I know for myself the relationship I have with my animals contributes hugely towards my well-being, it's something I can't explain, but from a young age, I've always felt drawn to animals. Also, the relationship we have with our environment, God, or nature. And the relationship we even have towards our own health.

When we consider the rather deep question, 'who am I.' that was mentioned earlier, it can raise much contemplation, but I'd encourage you to really give it some thought, we may be a wife, husband, boyfriend, girlfriend, mother, father, son, daughter, employee, employer, but underneath all that – *who am I* . I think we can't really answer that question without reflecting on our values, what are the values we live by, now they may be values that have been imposed on us by our culture, the society in which we belong. Examples of such are ' I must achieve', 'I must be beautiful', 'I must be thin,' 'I must have the latest fashions'…….etc. in order to be accepted. But I'm suggesting we consider going a little bit deeper and thinking what is my moral code that feels right to me. Not one that has been imposed, that might be the one that feels right, but if not, if we truly be still and tune in to the bit of us that is the real essence of us, what comes up?

I'd like to invite you to write down anything that comes to mind that seems to capture your *true* values. I'd then invite you to think about how true you live your life according to your values. Is there a good fit? Are your values at odds with the life you are living? How does that effect your wellbeing?

These are interesting questions, and I don't expect you to arrive at a quick answer, but sometimes the space in between what our true values are and the life we are living can be a cause for discomfort and can grate and jar. However, I do believe there are always compromises, I guess the question is how much is the compromise contributing to our dis-ease, or lack of well-being?

Although in some ways this has been a whistle stop tour, I would invite you to take what you need from this short book, at this time, to help you on your own unique wellbeing path, but I'd also encourage you to revisit the book, when you need to. This may be when something isn't quite working for you in your life, if you re-read

the chapter, chapters you're most drawn to, I
would suggest there may be something in
there that might shed some light on the matter.

I remember reading a book some years ago
that I just couldn't get on with at all, it was like it
was written in a foreign language, I returned to
the book a few years later and it made such
perfect sense to me, it was like it had been
written for me. Whilst I enjoyed the book
immensely, I was left feeling slightly annoyed,
why couldn't I have understood it a couple of
years ago, the answer was because I wasn't
ready to hear it!

Like the title of the book, wellbeing, pure and
simple, in some ways it is, but in some ways, it
isn't. I would say it takes deliberate effort to
stay well and this will be on a continuum for
most of us.

This book also isn't a substitute for contacting
a professional, if you feel you would like to talk
to someone to explore any of the issues that
have come up for you further, then I would

encourage you to do so. Below are some ideas of where to get support.

Talk to your G.P

Refer yourself to your local IAPT service, you will usually find information around how to do this on an internet search.

Here is a link to find a Counsellor/therapist

www.bacp.co.uk

Also

www.counsellingdirectory.co.uk

Here is a link to find a Cognitive Behavioural Therapist, although Cognitive Behavioural therapists may also be found on the above website.

www.babcp.co.uk

Another link to find a talking therapist.

www.ukcp.co.uk

To look for a shamanic healer

www.shamanic-practitioners.co.uk

ABOUT THE AUTHOR

Nic Hartshorne is an Integrative Relational Therapist and Supervisor working in Private Practice and the NHS.   Nic has many years' experience working with clients.